Southern Keto Cookbook

Free Gift Included

As part of our commitment to making sure you live a healthy lifestyle, we have included a free e-book in the link below. This book gives you a list of foods that you incorporate into your daily life to lose weight and live healthier. The link to the gift is below:

http://36potentfoodstoloseweightandlivehealthy.gr8.com

Disclaimer

Copyright © 2020

All Rights Reserved.

No part of this book can be transmitted or reproduced in any form including print, electronic, photocopying, scanning, mechanical or recording without prior written permission from the author.

While the author has taken utmost efforts to ensure the accuracy of the written content, all readers are advised to follow information mentioned herein at their own risk. The author cannot be held responsible for any personal or commercial damage caused by information. All readers are encouraged to seek professional advice when needed. This book is not written by a medical doctor and does not provide cures for any diseases. Please consult a professional doctor if you are sick.

Table of Contents

FREE GIFT INCLUDED 2

DISCLAIMER 3

TABLE OF CONTENTS 5

INTRODUCTION 9

FRIED CHICKEN RECIPES 12

    FRIED CHICKEN WITH ALMOND FLOUR AND PARMESAN 12

    KETO FRIED CHICKEN IN OVEN 14

    SOUTHERN FRIED CHICKEN TENDERS 16

    SOUTHERN FRIED CHICKEN WITH COCONUT FLOUR 18

    SOUTHERN STYLE FRIED CHICKEN WITH BUTTERMILK 19

CAJUN RECIPES 21

    CAJUN SEASONING 21

    CAJUN CAULIFLOWER MINI DOGS 22

    CAJUN JAMBALAYA 24

    CAJUN CHICKEN TACOS 26

    CAJUN CHICKEN, SAUSAGE, AND VEGETABLE SKILLET 28

    CAJUN CHICKEN PASTA 30

    KETO CAJUN CHICKEN NUGGETS 33

    CAJUN CAULIFLOWER HASH 35

    CAJUN CAULIFLOWER RICE 37

    BLACKENED CAJUN MAHI MAHI 38

    BLACKENED SALMON WITH CAJUN ZOODLES 40

    CAJUN SALMON FILLETS WITH SHRIMP & CREAM SAUCE 42

KETO WAFFLE RECIPES 44

    KETO WAFFLES 44

    CHOCOLATE WAFFLES 46

- Chocolate Hazelnut Protein Waffles 48
- Chocolate Chip Waffles 50
- Strawberry Shortcake Waffle 52
- Keto Vegan Pumpkin Waffle 54
- Cauliflower Hash Brown Waffles 55
- Cheese and Ham Waffles 57
- Okra Fritter Cheese Waffle 59
- Buffalo Chicken Waffle 61
- Keto Peanut Butter Cup Waffle 62

GRITS AND BISCUITS 64

- Breakfast Grits 64
- Keto Cheese Grits 66
- Comforting Keto Grits 67
- Keto Shrimp and Cauliflower "Grits" 68
- Breakfast Biscuit with Coconut Flour 70
- Keto Biscuits 71
- **Stuffed Breakfast Biscuits** 72
- Southern Style Fluffy Biscuits 74
- Southern Biscuits and Gravy 76

LOWCOUNTRY RECIPES 78

- Keto Country Gravy 78
- Chicken Shrimp Gumbo with Sausage 79
- Crab Deviled Eggs 81
- Lowcountry Seafood Boil 82
- Keto Mississippi Roast 84
- Keto Creamy Crab Soup 86
- Southern Summer Tomato Pie 87
- Cajun Shrimp Boil 89
- Lowcountry-style Shrimp and Grits 90
- Low Country Shrimp Frittata 93
- Keto Dogs 95

FLORIBBEAN RECIPES 97

- Jamaican-Style Brown Chicken Stew 97
- Jamaican Callaloo 99
- Callaloo and Saltfish 101
- Jerk Prawns 102
- Grilled Hogfish Snapper with Old Bay Compound Butter 104
- Low Carb Keto Arroz Con Pollo (Spanish rice with Chicken) 105
- Ajiaco 107
- Jerk Chicken 108
- Jerk Chicken Salad 110
- Jamaican Chicken Curry 111
- Jamaican Meat Pies or Patties 113
- Keto Cuban Pork (Lechón) 116
- Keto Cuban Sliders 118
- Keto Cuban Cups 119
- Puerto Rican Chicken 120
- Caribbean Callaloo Soup 122
- Caribbean Callaloo and Crab 124

SOUTHERN DESSERT RECIPES 126

- Southern Butter Keto Pound Cake 126
- **Chocolate Cake** 128
- Keto Southern Coconut Pecan Cake 130
- Pumpkin Pie 133
- Keto Apple Pie 135
- Vegan Keto Chocolate Pie 138
- Berry Crisp 140
- Blackberry Cobbler 141
- Brownies 143
- Lime Fluff 145
- Keto Churros 147

CONCLUSION 149

Introduction

The Southern culture came into existence when British soldiers stepped into Jamestown, Virginia with a few pigs in the year 1607. The locals in the area, the Powhatan Indians, took time to share knowledge of the spices they used to cook their food. It was only after a few years that the Powhatan Indians guided the British through the blossoming botanicals. They revealed their secrets about the new flavors hidden in the land. Over time, people from other countries came to Virginia, and the food prepared in this Southern state soon changed. It became a mixture of domestic and foreign traditions and food. The Southern cuisine is one of the most diverse and traditional styles of cooking that has passed through generations. Our objective is not to trace the history of this cuisine, but to look at the some of the classic Southern dishes that are keto-friendly.

Most people avoid the Southern diet since it is not very healthy, but this is not the case with all the dishes. Like every cuisine, there are some dishes in the Southern diet that are healthy. You can also use substitute ingredients that are low-carb. When you follow the ketogenic diet, you need to consume meals that are low-carb and high fat. These dishes should, however, include a moderate amount of protein. When you reduce your intake of carbohydrates, your body will need to look for an alternative means to produce energy since the glucose levels in your body will decrease. The only option your body has is to target the stored fat and the fat in food to produce energy. When your body breaks the fat down into ketones, your body will shift into the metabolic state called ketosis. When your body begins to burn fat, you lose weight faster. It is for this reason that people lose weight quickly when they follow the ketogenic diet. The ketogenic diet has amazing benefits for your overall health.

The ketogenic diet in essence is a diet that will force the body to release ketones into the bloodstream. When your body reaches the metabolic state called ketosis, the cells will start using these ketone bodies to produce energy until you consume carbohydrates again. Remember that the ketogenic diet is a highly individualized process. This means that you may need to follow a more restricted diet if you want to produce more ketones.

You may now wonder how one can consume Southern dishes when they are on the ketogenic diet since this cuisine is very high in carbohydrates, greasy and honestly, not very good for your heart. Having said that, it is possible for you to prepare a healthy Southern meal that will taste extremely good. If you are craving a Southern meal, you should pick the recipes in this book. These recipes are yummy, simple and low-carb versions of a Southern dish. This book has tasty meal ideas and recipes that will curb your cravings and help you stick to a healthy meal plan. You will find recipes from fried chicken to Mississippi mud pie and more. All you need to remember is that you can follow a ketogenic diet without worrying about the cuisine you follow. You must reduce your carbohydrate intake to ensure that your body produces more ketones. This is the only way you can lose weight.

If you are craving for some good 'ole southern comfort food, you have come to the right place. This book has the best recipes that you can use to curb your Southern craving. The recipes in this book are keto-friendly which means that they are low-carb and have very little sugar. The food in this book will fit your healthy diet, and you can eat without feeling guilty. This is perfect isn't it?

Thank you for purchasing this book. I hope you enjoy the delicious recipes and continue to follow the ketogenic diet.

This book is not written by a medical doctor and does not provide cures for any diseases. Please consult a professional doctor if you are looking to make significant changes to your diet.

Fried Chicken Recipes

Fried Chicken with Almond Flour and Parmesan

Serves: 3

Ingredients:

- 1 pound chicken thigh fillets, cut each fillet into 3 equal pieces
- 1 teaspoon celery salt
- ½ teaspoon dried oregano
- ½ teaspoon garlic powder
- ¼ teaspoon chili powder
- 1 tablespoon heavy cream
- 1 small egg
- ¼ cup finely grated Parmesan cheese
- ¼ cup almond meal

Directions:

1. Place chicken in a bowl.
2. Mix together garlic powder, chili powder, celery salt and oregano in a bowl and sprinkle over the chicken. Toss well set aside for 30 minutes.
3. In the meantime, add egg and cream into a bowl and whisk well.
4. Add almond flour and Parmesan cheese into a shallow bowl.

5. Set up the deep fryer and let it heat to 355° F.
6. First dip the chicken pieces in egg mixture, one at a time and then dredge in the almond flour mixture and place on a tray.
7. Fry the chicken in the deep fryer in batches, until golden brown in color or until the chicken is cooked through. Remove the chicken and place on a plate lined with paper towels.
8. Serve hot.

Keto Fried Chicken in Oven

Serves: 6

Ingredients:

- 2 ounces pork rinds, crushed
- ½ teaspoon sea salt
- ½ teaspoon dried oregano
- ½ teaspoon smoked paprika
- ¾ teaspoon dried thyme
- ½ teaspoon pepper
- ¼ teaspoon garlic powder
- 6 legs and thighs bone-in chicken pieces, skinless
- 1 ounce mayonnaise
- 1 small egg
- 1 ½ tablespoons Dijon mustard

Directions:

1. Add pork rinds, salt and all the spices into a shallow bowl and stir until well combined.
2. Add egg, Dijon mustard and mayonnaise into a bowl and whisk well.
3. Place a wire rack on a baking sheet.
4. First dip the chicken pieces in the egg mixture, one at a time and then dredge in the pork rind mixture and place on the wire rack.
5. Bake in a preheated oven at 400° F for about 40 minutes or until baked through.

Southern Fried Chicken Tenders

Serves: 2

Ingredients:

- 2 chicken breasts
- 1 small egg, beaten
- 2.5 ounces almond flour
- 1 teaspoon cayenne pepper
- 1 teaspoon garlic powder
- 1 teaspoon onion salt
- 1 teaspoon dried mixed herbs
- ½ teaspoon pepper
- ½ teaspoon salt

Directions:

1. Place cayenne pepper, garlic powder, onion salt, herbs, salt and pepper in a bowl and stir until well combined.
2. Rub this mixture into the chicken pieces. Place in a bowl. Cover and chill for 2 – 8 hours.
3. First dip the chicken pieces in the egg, one at a time and then dredge in the almond flour and place on a tray.
4. Set up the deep fryer and let it heat to 355° F.
5. Fry the chicken in the deep fryer in batches until golden brown in color or until the chicken is cooked through. Remove the chicken and place on a plate lined with paper towels.
6. Serve hot.

Southern Fried Chicken with Coconut Flour

Serves: 5 – 6

Ingredients:

- 2 ½ pounds chicken leg quarters
- ½ teaspoon pepper
- ½ teaspoon salt
- ½ teaspoon paprika
- ½ teaspoon garlic powder
- ½ cup coconut flour
- Oil to fry, as required

Directions:

1. Add garlic powder, salt, pepper and paprika in a bowl and stir. Rub this mixture into the chicken pieces. Place in a bowl. Cover and chill for 2 – 8 hours.
2. Sprinkle coconut flour on the chicken and toss well.
3. Place a deep, heavy bottomed pan over medium heat. Add enough oil to cover the bottom of the pan (2 inches of the height of the pan). When the oil is heated, add chicken in batches.
4. Fry until golden brown or until cooked through.
5. Remove the chicken with a slotted spoon and place on a plate lined with paper towels.
6. Serve hot.

Southern Style Fried Chicken with Buttermilk

Serves: 5 – 6

Ingredients:

- ¾ cup buttermilk
- 2 ½ pounds chicken, cut into 5 – 6 pieces
- 2 teaspoon kosher salt
- ¾ teaspoon pepper
- ½ teaspoon red pepper flakes or to taste
- ¼ teaspoon dried fennel
- ¼ teaspoon chili powder or to taste
- 1 teaspoons dried Italian herbs
- ½ package Sazon
- ¼ teaspoon onion powder
- ¼ teaspoon garlic powder
- ¼ teaspoon Cajun seasoning
- 1 cup almond flour
- ½ cup coconut flour
- Peanut oil to fry, as required

Directions:

1. Place chicken in a bowl. Pour buttermilk over it. Set aside for 30 minutes.
2. Add spices and salt and mix well.
3. Sprinkle coconut flour and almond flour over the chicken and mix until chicken is well coated in the batter. Remove the chicken pieces and shake to drop off excess batter.

4. Place a deep, heavy bottomed pan over medium heat. Add enough oil to cover the bottom of the pan (2 inches of the height of the pan). When the oil is heated, add chicken in batches.
5. Fry until golden brown or until cooked through.
6. Remove the chicken with a slotted spoon and place on a plate lined with paper towels.
7. Serve hot.

Cajun Recipes

Cajun Seasoning

Makes: About 1 ½ cups

Ingredients:

- 6 tablespoons paprika
- 4 tablespoons garlic powder
- 2 tablespoons ground white pepper
- 2 tablespoons ground black pepper
- 2 tablespoons dried oregano
- 2 tablespoons onion powder
- 2 tablespoons cayenne pepper
- 4 tablespoons fine kosher salt
- 1 tablespoon dried thyme
- 1 tablespoon salt

Directions:

1. Add all the ingredients into a jar and stir until well incorporated.
2. Seal the jar and store in a cool and dry place.
3. Use as required.

Cajun Cauliflower Mini Dogs

Serves: 12

Ingredients:

- 24 mini Cajun spiced sausages
- ½ cup coconut flour
- 3 tablespoons coconut oil or butter, melted
- 1 teaspoon ground mustard
- Salt to taste
- 1-2 jalapeños, minced (optional)
- 2 cups grated cauliflower, grated to rice like texture
- 4 large eggs, beaten
- ½ cup grated cheese of your choice
- 1 teaspoon baking soda mixed with 2 teaspoons apple cider vinegar
- 2 tablespoons hot sauce (optional)
- ½ teaspoon smoked paprika
- ¼ teaspoon chili powder

To serve: Optional

- Hot sauce
- Mustard

Directions:

1. Add coconut flour, butter, salt jalapeños, cauliflower, eggs, cheese, baking soda mixture, hot sauce, paprika and chili powder into a bowl and mix well.

2. Divide the mixture into 24 portions. Place one portion on your palm and flatten it. Place a mini sausage in the center and bring the edges together to cover the hot dogs from all the sides. Place on a baking sheet lined with parchment paper.
3. Bake in a preheated oven at 400° F for about 20-25 minutes until top is brown and firm.
4. Remove from the oven. Cool for a few minutes. Chop into 2 if desired and serve.
5. Serve with mustard and hot sauce if desired.

Cajun Jambalaya

Serves: 10

Ingredients:

- 6 tablespoons olive oil
- 2 cups diced red onion
- 16 ounces smoked turkey sausage, chopped into chunks
- 2 pounds chicken breast, chopped into chunks
- 16 ounces raw jumbo shrimp, peeled, deveined
- 4 cloves garlic, peeled, minced
- 2 green bell peppers, diced
- 2 cups quartered cherry tomatoes
- 6 tablespoons tomato paste
- 16 ounces tomato sauce
- 3 cups low sodium chicken broth
- 4 cups cauliflower rice
- 4 bay leaves
- 6 tablespoons Cajun seasoning
- Salt to taste
- 1 green onion, thinly sliced, to garnish

Directions:

1. To make cauliflower rice, you can buy from the store or make it at home. To make it at home, you can either grate the cauliflower to rice like texture. You can also place cauliflower florets in the food processor and pulse until rice like in texture.

2. Squeeze the cauliflower of excess moisture if desired.
3. Place a soup pot over medium heat. Add oil. When the oil is heated, add garlic and onions and sauté until light brown.
4. Stir in the sausage and chicken and cook until the chicken is not pink anymore.
5. Stir in celery, bell pepper and tomatoes. Cook for a minute.
6. Stir in Cajun seasoning and tomato sauce. Simmer for a few minutes.
7. Add cauliflower rice and shrimp and cook for 3 – 4 minutes.
8. Stir in the broth, salt, pepper, bay leaves and tomato paste. Lower the heat to low heat.
9. Cover and cook for 15 – 20 minutes or until chicken is cooked through. Turn off the heat.
10. Uncover and let the jambalaya sit for 10 -15 minutes.
11. Taste and adjust the seasonings if required.
12. Ladle into bowls. Sprinkle green onions on top and serve.

Cajun Chicken Tacos

Serves: 4

Ingredients:

- 2 packages chicken thighs (14.1 ounces each), diced
- Juice of a lime
- 2 tablespoons chopped fresh oregano or 1 teaspoon dried oregano
- 2 tablespoons chopped fresh thyme or 1 teaspoon dried thyme
- 1 teaspoon paprika
- 4 tablespoons ghee or butter
- Salt to taste
- Pepper to taste
- 1 medium red onion, finely chopped
- 4 cloves garlic, smashed
- ½ teaspoon cayenne pepper
- 4 ounces fresh full fat cream or coconut milk
- 4 small heads lettuce, separate the leaves

Directions:

1. Add chicken thighs, garlic, thyme, oregano, paprika, pepper, salt, lime juice and cayenne pepper into a bowl and toss well. You can add the Cajun seasoning instead of these spices.
2. Place a large skillet over medium heat. Add ghee. When ghee melts, add onions and sauté until golden brown.

3. Add the chicken along with the spice mixture and sauté until the chicken is cooked through.
4. Stir in the cream and cook for a couple of minutes. Turn off the heat.
5. Place the lettuce leaves on a large serving platter.
6. Divide the chicken among the leaves and serve.

Cajun Chicken, Sausage, and Vegetable Skillet

Serves: 8

Ingredients:

- 2 tablespoons olive oil
- 16 ounces Andouille sausage, cut into medium size pieces
- 2 medium green bell peppers, diced
- 2 medium red bell peppers, diced
- 2 cups chopped red onions
- 2 medium zucchinis, cut into small pieces
- 2 stalks celery, sliced
- 2 teaspoons thyme
- 2 teaspoons red pepper (optional)
- 2 chicken breasts, skinless, cut into cubes
- 1 tablespoon Cajun seasoning or more to taste
- Salt to taste
- Pepper to taste

Directions:

1. Add sausage and chicken into a large bowl and toss well.
2. Add bell peppers, onion, zucchini and celery into another bowl and toss well.
3. Pour a tablespoon of oil into each bowl and toss well. Sprinkle salt and pepper in each bowl. Divide the Cajun seasoning among the bowls and toss well.

4. Place a large skillet over medium-high heat. Transfer the chicken and sausage mixture into the skillet and cook until the chicken is not pink anymore.
5. Remove with a slotted spoon and place in a bowl.
6. Transfer the vegetables from the bowl into the skillet and cook until tender.
7. Add the chicken and sausage back into the skillet and mix well.
8. Serve hot.

Cajun Chicken Pasta

Serves: 8

Ingredients:

<u>For Cajun chicken:</u>

- 4 tablespoons butter, divided
- 4 teaspoons Cajun seasoning or to taste, divided
- 2 teaspoons minced garlic
- ½ cup chopped scallions
- 1 cup chicken broth
- 1 cup shredded Monterey Jack cheese
- ½ cup chopped cilantro
- 2 pounds chicken cutlets
- 1 cup chopped tomatoes
- ½ cup dry white wine
- ½ cup heavy whipping cream
- 2 ounces cream cheese
- Salt to taste
- Pepper to taste

<u>For the fettuccine pasta:</u>

- 16 eggs
- ½ teaspoon salt or to taste
- ½ teaspoon pepper or to taste
- 8 ounces cream cheese
- ½ teaspoon garlic powder

Directions:

1. For Cajun chicken: Sprinkle 2 teaspoons Cajun seasoning all over the chicken.
2. Place a skillet over medium heat. Add 2 tablespoons butter. When butter melts, add chicken and cook for 2 minutes. Flip sides and cook for another 2 – 3 minutes or until cooked inside.
3. Take out the chicken and place on a plate.
4. Add 2 tablespoons butter. When butter melts, add garlic and sauté until aromatic.
5. Stir in the tomatoes and cook for a couple of minutes. Next add the wine and simmer for a couple of minutes.
6. Stir in the 2 teaspoons Cajun seasoning and broth and simmer for 5 – 6 minutes.
7. Add cream cheese, cream and cheese and stir constantly until thick.
8. Stir in cilantro and scallions. Turn off the heat.
9. For fettuccine: Add all the ingredients for fettuccine into a blender and blend until smooth. Set aside for 5 minutes.
10. Grease a large rimmed baking sheet with some cooking spray. Place a sheet of parchment paper on it. Use 2 baking sheets if required.
11. Pour the egg mixture into the baking sheet.
12. Bake in a preheated oven at 325° F for about 8 – 10 minutes or until eggs are just cooked.
13. Remove the baking sheet from the oven and let it rest for 5 minutes.
14. Loosen the pasta from the baking sheet. Cut into 1/8 inch wide slices.

15. Serve chicken with gravy over pasta.

Keto Cajun Chicken Nuggets

Serves: 8

Ingredients:

- 4 chicken breasts, cut into nugget size
- 2 – 6 cups milk of your choice
- 3 – 4 tablespoons Cajun seasoning or more if required
- 6 ounces pork rinds, ground
- 6 eggs
- Cayenne pepper to taste (optional)
- Paprika to taste (optional)
- Canola oil or vegetable oil, as required

Directions:

1. Add eggs into a bowl and whisk well. Add some milk and a generous amount of Cajun seasoning. Mix well.
2. Sprinkle paprika, cayenne pepper and some Cajun seasoning on the nuggets.
3. Place chicken in the bowl of egg mixture. The nuggets should be covered in milk. So add milk accordingly. Let it marinate for 10 minutes.
4. Add pork rinds and a generous amount of Cajun seasoning into a Ziploc bag. Take out only the nuggets from the milk and place in the Ziploc bag. Shake the bag around so that the nuggets are well coated with the pork rinds. Set aside for 10 minutes.

5. Place a pan over medium heat. Add enough oil to cover the bottom of the pan by at least 2 inches.
6. When the oil is well heated but not smoking, add some nuggets. The nuggets should be covered in oil. Do not overcrowd. Lower the heat to low heat and cook until golden brown. When done, the nuggets will float on top.
7. Remove with a slotted spoon and place on a plate lined with paper towels.
8. Fry the remaining nuggets similarly.
9. You can also bake it in an oven if you do not prefer fried.

Cajun Cauliflower Hash

Serves: 4

Ingredients:

- 4 tablespoons olive oil or ghee
- 4 tablespoons minced garlic
- 2 teaspoons Cajun seasoning or more to taste + extra to garnish
- 1 green pepper, chopped into ¼ inch pieces
- 1 onion, chopped into ¼ inch pieces
- 2 pounds frozen cauliflower, steamed, chopped into small pieces, squeezed of excess moisture
- 16 ounces shaved red pastrami, chopped into 1 inch slices

To serve:

- 4 eggs, cooked sunny side up

Directions:

1. Place a skillet over medium heat. Add oil. When the oil is heated, add onions and cook until onions are translucent.
2. Add garlic and sauté for a couple of minutes until the garlic is fragrant.
3. Add cauliflower and sauté until light brown and crisp.
4. Stir in the Cajun seasoning.
5. Add pastrami and green pepper. Heat thoroughly.
6. Transfer into 4 serving bowls.

7. Top with eggs. Sprinkle some more Cajun seasoning on top and serve.

Cajun Cauliflower Rice

Serves: 8

Ingredients:

- 2 green bell pepper, diced
- 4 teaspoons minced garlic
- 2 medium onions, diced
- 24 ounces Andouille sausage, sliced
- 4 tablespoons Cajun seasoning
- 8 cups frozen cauliflower rice
- Salt to taste
- Pepper to taste
- 2 tablespoons avocado oil or any other oil
- A handful fresh parsley, chopped, to garnish

Directions:

1. Place a large skillet or wok over medium-high heat.
2. Add oil. When the oil is heated, add garlic, onion and bell pepper and sauté until slightly tender.
3. Stir the sausages and cook until light brown.
4. Stir in the seasonings and cauliflower rice. When the rice is well heated, turn off the heat.
5. Sprinkle parsley on top and serve.

Blackened Cajun Mahi Mahi

Serves: 4

Ingredients:

For blackened Cajun spice dry rub:

- 2 teaspoons dried parsley
- 2 teaspoons dried thyme
- 2 teaspoons dried oregano
- 1 teaspoon cayenne pepper
- 2 teaspoons smoked paprika
- 1 teaspoon garlic powder
- 1 teaspoon onion powder
- 1 teaspoon pepper powder
- 1 teaspoon salt

For blackened Cajun Mahi Mahi:

- 4 Mahi Mahi fish fillets (6 ounces each)
- 2 avocadoes, peeled, pitted, sliced
- 2 tablespoons coconut oil
- Lime wedges to serve

Directions:

1. To make blackened Cajun spice dry rub: Add all the ingredients for the Cajun spice rub into a wide shallow bowl. Mix well.

2. Coat fillets in the spice rub.
3. Place a large skillet over medium high heat. Add oil. When the oil, place 2-3 fillets or as many as can fit in the pan. Cook the remaining in batches.
4. Cook for 3-4 minutes on each side or until the fish flakes easily when pierced with a fork.
5. Remove on to a plate.
6. Place avocado slices on top. Serve with lime wedges.

Blackened Salmon with Cajun Zoodles

Serves: 4

Ingredients:

- 8 medium zucchini, trimmed
- 2 red bell peppers, finely diced
- 8 tablespoons butter or ghee, divided
- 2 teaspoons salt or to taste
- 4 cloves garlic, crushed
- 1 ½ pounds wild caught salmon
- 2 tablespoons Cajun seasoning or to taste
- Lemon wedges to serve

Directions:

1. Make noodles of the zucchini using a spiralizer or a julienne noodles.
2. Spread the noodles on a kitchen towel. Season with a teaspoon of salt. Let it sit for 20 – 30 minutes. Rinse well and place in a colander. Dry the zucchini noodles with a dry kitchen towel.
3. Season one side of the fillets with a little salt. Sprinkle a generous amount of Cajun seasoning over the fillets.
4. Flip sides and sprinkle salt on the other side. Sprinkle a generous amount of Cajun seasoning over the fillets.
5. Place a large skillet over medium-high heat. Add 4 tablespoons butter. When butter melts, place salmon in the pan and cook for 2 minutes. Flip sides and cook the

other side for 2 minutes or until the fish flakes easily when pierced with a fork. Cook in batches if required.
6. Remove fish with a slotted spoon and place on a plate lined with parchment paper.
7. Add remaining butter into the skillet. When butter melts, add bell pepper and sauté for a couple of minutes.
8. Add noodles and garlic and toss well. Add salt if required and some more Cajun seasoning.
9. Turn off the heat. Divide noodles into individual serving plates. Place salmon on top. Serve with lemon wedges.

Cajun Salmon Fillets with Shrimp & Cream Sauce

Serves: 8

Ingredients:

- 2 pounds salmon fillets
- 2 tablespoons olive oil
- 1 cup red bell pepper, diced
- 2 cups heavy cream
- 4 tablespoons butter
- ½ cup diced shallots
- 1 pound baby shrimp
- 6 tablespoons Cajun seasoning

Directions:

1. Season the fish on both the sides with 2 tablespoons of seasoning.
2. Place a skillet over medium-high heat. Add oil. When the oil is heated, place the fish in the pan and cook for 2 – 3 minutes. Flip sides and cook the other side for 2 – 3 minutes.
3. Remove fish with a slotted spoon and place on a plate.
4. Add 2 tablespoons butter. When butter melts, add shallots and cook until light brown.
5. Stir in the red pepper and sauté for a minutes.
6. Add cream, 3 tablespoons Cajun seasoning and salt and cook for a couple of minutes.

7. Stir in the shrimp. Let it come to a simmer. Turn off the heat.
8. Divide the fish into serving plates. Spoon shrimp with gravy over the fish and serve.

Keto Waffle Recipes

Keto Waffles

Serves: 10

Ingredients:

- 10 eggs, separated
- 8-10 tablespoons granulated stevia or erythritol, or to taste
- 2 – 4 teaspoons vanilla
- 9 ounces butter, melted
- 1/3 cup full fat milk
- ½ cup coconut flour
- 2 teaspoons baking powder
- Ghee or butter, to grease

Directions:

1. Beat the egg whites with an electric hand mixer until stiff peaks are formed. Set aside.
2. Beat the yolks. Add coconut flour and stevia and whisk until smooth and free from lumps.
3. Drizzle melted butter and whisk until smooth.
4. Whisk in the milk and vanilla. Whisk until smooth.
5. Add egg whites, a little at a time and fold gently. .
6. Plug in the waffle maker and let it preheat to medium-high heat.

7. Grease the waffle maker with ghee. Pour about ¼ cup of batter into the waffle maker.
8. Close the lid and cook until crisp and brown.
9. Remove the waffle and place on a baking sheet in an oven to keep warm.
10. Repeat steps 7 – 9 and make the remaining waffles.
11. Serve with a topping of your choice like berries, whipped cream, etc. if desired.

Chocolate Waffles

Serves: 10

Ingredients:

- 10 eggs, separated
- 1.8 ounces cocoa, unsweetened
- 2 teaspoon baking powder
- 6 tablespoons full fat milk or cream
- 7.7 ounces butter, melted
- 8 tablespoons coconut flour
- 8 tablespoons granulated sweetener of your choice
- 4 teaspoons vanilla extract
- Butter or ghee, to grease

Directions:

1. Beat the whites with an electric hand mixer until stiff peaks are formed.
2. Add coconut flour, sweetener, cocoa and baking powder into the bowl of yolks. Whisk well.
3. Drizzle melted butter and whisk until smooth.
4. Whisk in the milk and vanilla. Whisk until smooth.
5. Add egg whites, a little at a time and fold gently.
6. Plug in the waffle maker and let it preheat to medium-high heat.
7. Grease the waffle maker with ghee. Pour about ¼ cup of batter into the waffle maker.
8. Close the lid and cook until crisp and brown.

9. Remove the waffle and place on a baking sheet in an oven to keep warm.
10. Repeat steps 7 – 9 and make the remaining waffles.
11. Serve with toppings of your choice like berries, whipped cream, sugar-free chocolate syrup etc. if desired

Chocolate Hazelnut Protein Waffles

Serves: 12 thick waffles or 16 thinner waffles

Ingredients:

- 2 cups hazelnut meal
- ¼ cup cocoa powder
- 1 cup chocolate protein powder
- ¼ cup coconut flour
- 8 large eggs
- 6 tablespoons hazelnut oil
- 6 tablespoons swerve sweetener or granulated erythritol
- ½ teaspoon stevia extract
- 2/3 cup full fat Greek yogurt
- A little melted ghee for greasing

Directions:

1. Add hazelnut meal, cocoa, protein powder, coconut flour and swerve into a large bowl and mix well.
2. Add eggs, yogurt, hazelnut oil, hazelnut extract and stevia and whisk until smooth and free from lumps.
3. Plug in the waffle maker and let it preheat to medium-high heat.
4. Grease the waffle maker with ghee. Pour about ¼ cup of batter into the waffle maker.
5. Close the lid and cook until crisp and brown.
6. Remove the waffle and place on a baking sheet in an oven to keep warm.

7. Repeat steps 4 – 6 and make the remaining waffles.
8. Serve with toppings of your choice like chopped hazelnuts, whipped cream, sugar-free syrup etc. if desired.

Chocolate Chip Waffles

Serves: 4

Ingredients:

- 4 scoops keto friendly vanilla protein powder, unsweetened
- 4 tablespoons butter, melted
- 3.5 ounces sugar-free chocolate chips or cacao nibs
- 4 large eggs, separated
- ¼ teaspoon Himalayan pink salt
- 1 cup sugar-free maple syrup
- Butter to serve
- Ghee, to grease

Directions:

1. Beat the whites with an electric hand mixer until stiff peaks are formed.
2. Add protein powder, butter and yolks into a bowl and stir until well combined.
3. Add whites and fold gently. Stir in cacao nibs and salt.
4. Plug in the waffle maker and let it preheat to medium-high heat.
5. Grease the waffle maker with ghee. Pour about ¼ cup of batter into the waffle maker.
6. Close the lid and cook until crisp and brown.
7. Remove the waffle and place on a baking sheet in an oven to keep warm.

8. Repeat steps 5 – 7 and make the remaining waffles.
9. Top with sugar-free maple syrup and some butter and serve.

Strawberry Shortcake Waffle

Serves: 2

Ingredients:

- 2 eggs
- 2 teaspoons coconut flour
- 1 teaspoon cake batter extract
- 2 tablespoons heavy whipping cream
- 4 tablespoons swerve or erythritol
- ½ teaspoon baking powder
- Butter or ghee, to grease

To serve:

- Whipped cream
- Strawberry slices
- Swerve confectioners

Directions:

1. Plug in the waffle maker and let it preheat to medium-high heat.
2. Add eggs into a bowl and whisk with a fork.
3. Add rest of the ingredients and stir until well combined.
4. Grease the waffle maker with ghee. Pour half the batter into the waffle maker.
5. Close the lid and cook until crisp and brown.
6. Remove the waffle and place on a baking sheet in an oven to keep warm.

7. Repeat steps 4 – 6 and make the remaining waffle.
8. Sprinkle some swerve confectioners. Scatter strawberries on top and serve with whipped cream.

Keto Vegan Pumpkin Waffle

Serves: 2

Ingredients:

- 2 tablespoons coconut cream
- 12 tablespoons almond flour
- 4 tablespoons pumpkin puree
- 2 flax eggs (2 tablespoons flaxseeds mixed with 5 tablespoons water and set aside for 10 – 12 minutes)
- ½ teaspoon xanthan gum
- 4 tablespoons Sukrin Gold
- 2 teaspoons pumpkin pie spice
- Oil, to grease

Directions:

1. Plug in the waffle maker and let it preheat to medium-high heat.
2. Add all the ingredients into a bowl and whisk into a thick batter.
3. Grease the waffle maker with oil. Pour half the batter into the waffle maker.
4. Close the lid and cook until crisp and brown.
5. Remove the waffle and place on a baking sheet in an oven to keep warm.
6. Repeat steps 3 – 5 and make the remaining waffle.

Cauliflower Hash Brown Waffles

Serves: 6

Ingredients:

- 2 medium heads cauliflower, grated
- 2 large bunches scallions, finely chopped
- 4 tablespoons olive oil + extra to grease
- Salt to taste
- Pepper to taste
- 4 eggs
- 16 ounces ham, cubed
- 5-6 tablespoons shredded cheddar cheese, (optional)
- A handful of fresh herbs of your choice, chopped to garnish
- Oil, to grease

Directions:

1. Add cauliflower, scallions, oil, salt, pepper, eggs, ham and cheese if using into a bowl and mix well.
2. Grease a waffle iron generously with oil and let it preheat to medium- high heat.
3. Pour about ¼ cup of batter into the waffle maker.
4. Close the lid and cook until crisp and brown.

5. Remove the waffle and place on a baking sheet in an oven to keep warm.
6. Repeat steps 5 – 7 and make the remaining waffles.
7. Garnish with herbs and serve with sour cream or coconut milk yogurt or any other keto friendly toppings if desired.

Cheese and Ham Waffles

Serves: 4

Ingredients:

- 8 large eggs
- 2 teaspoons baking powder
- 1 teaspoon sea salt
- 2 ounces cheddar cheese, finely grated
- A handful fresh basil, finely chopped
- 4 scoops unflavored whey protein powder
- 12 tablespoons melted butter
- ½ teaspoon paprika
- 2 ounces ham steak, finely chopped
- Ghee or butter, to grease

Directions:

1. Separate 4 eggs into yolks and whites into 2 mixing bowls.
2. Add the baking powder, sea salt, protein powder and melted butter into the bowl of yolks. Whisk until well incorporated.
3. Add grated cheese and chopped ham. Fold gently.
4. Add a pinch of salt to the bowl of the egg whites and whisk with the help of an electric hand mixer until stiff peaks form.
5. Mix half the whites mixture with the egg yolk mixture and fold well. Be extremely gentle when you are folding in the egg whites.

6. Once the egg yolks have aerated enough, add rest of the whites and fold gently.
7. Plug in the waffle maker and let it preheat to medium heat.
8. Grease the waffle maker with ghee. Pour about ¼ cup of batter into the waffle maker.
9. Close the lid and cook until crisp and brown.
10. Repeat steps 7 – 9 and make the remaining waffles.
11. As the waffles are cooking, cook 4 of the eggs, sunny sides up.
12. Arrange an egg on top of each waffle. Sprinkle some paprika and chopped basil over the egg.
13. Serve warm.

Okra Fritter Cheese Waffle

Serves: 4

Ingredients:

- 2 eggs
- 4 tablespoons heavy cream
- 1 teaspoon onion powder
- 8 tablespoons almond flour
- 2 tablespoons keto friendly mayonnaise
- 1 tablespoon creole seasoning
- 2 cups sliced okra, thaw if frozen
- ½ cup shredded mozzarella cheese or more if required
- Salt to taste
- Pepper to taste
- Ghee or butter, to grease

Directions:

1. Add eggs, cream, mayonnaise, salt, pepper and creole seasoning into a bowl and whisk well.
2. Add almond flour. Stir until well combined.
3. Stir in okra. Let the batter sit for 10 minutes.
4. Plug in the mini waffle maker and let it preheat to medium heat.
5. Grease the waffle maker with ghee.
6. Sprinkle a little mozzarella on the bottom of the waffle maker.

7. Spoon ¼ of the batter into the waffle maker. Close the waffle maker. Cook until golden brown.
8. Take out the chaffle when cooked and set aside on a plate. Let it sit for a couple of minutes.
9. Repeat steps 5 – 7 and make the remaining waffles.
10. Sprinkle a little salt on top and serve.

Buffalo Chicken Waffle

Serves: 2

Ingredients:

- 10 ounces canned or cooked chicken
- 10 tablespoons shredded cheddar cheese
- 2 eggs
- 4 tablespoons buffalo sauce
- 4 ounces cream cheese, softened
- Ghee or butter, to grease

Directions:

1. Beat eggs with a fork. Stir in cheddar cheese, chicken, cream cheese, buffalo and sauce.
2. Plug in the waffle maker and let it preheat to medium heat.
3. Grease the waffle maker with ghee.
4. Scatter some mozzarella cheese on the bottom of the waffle maker.
5. Spoon half the batter into the waffle maker. Scatter some mozzarella cheese on top of the batter. Close the waffle maker. Cook until crisp.
6. Repeat steps 3 – 5 and make the remaining waffle.

Keto Peanut Butter Cup Waffle

Serves: 4

Ingredients:

For waffles:

- 2 tablespoons heavy cream
- 2 tablespoons lakanato golden sweetener erythritol or swerve
- 1 teaspoon vanilla extract
- 2 eggs
- 2 teaspoons coconut flour
- 2 tablespoons unsweetened cocoa
- 1 teaspoon baking powder
- 1 teaspoon cake batter flavor extract
- Ghee or butter, to grease

For topping:

- 6 tablespoons natural peanut butter
- 4 tablespoons heavy cream
- 4 teaspoons lakanto powdered sweetener

Directions:

1. Plug in the mini waffle maker and let it preheat to medium heat.
2. Beat eggs with a fork. Add rest of the ingredients and whisk well. Let the batter sit for 3 to 4 minutes.

3. Grease the waffle maker with a little butter or ghee. Pour ¼ of the batter into the waffle maker. Close the waffle maker and cook until crisp.
4. Remove the waffle and set aside on a plate. Let it sit for a couple of minutes.
5. Repeat steps 3 – 5 and make the remaining waffles
6. To make peanut butter topping: Add peanut butter, cream and sweetener into a bowl and whisk well.
7. Spread peanut butter filling over the waffles and serve.

Grits and Biscuits

Breakfast Grits

Serves: 6

Ingredients:

- 24 ounces cauliflower, cut into florets
- 1 cup heavy whipping cream
- ½ teaspoon pepper or to taste
- ½ teaspoon salt or to taste
- 1 cup shredded sharp cheddar cheese
- 4 tablespoons unsalted butter
- 2 green onions, sliced

For toppings: Optional – use any

- Bacon slices, cooked, crumbled
- Crumbled feta cheese
- Eggs, fried or poached
- Chorizo, cooked until crisp

Directions:

1. Place cauliflower florets in the food processor bowl and process until rice like in texture.
2. Place a large pot over high heat. Add cauliflower and cook until slightly soft.

3. Stir in the cream and butter. Season with salt and pepper. Let it cook for about 4 minutes. Turn off the heat.
4. Blend a little of the cauliflower with an immersion blender until slightly smooth.
5. Ladle into bowls. Garnish with green onions and cheddar cheese and serve.

Keto Cheese Grits

Serves: 8

Ingredients:

- 2 cups super fine almond flour
- 1 teaspoon salt or to taste
- 2 cups water
- 1 cup shredded sharp cheddar cheese

Directions:

1. Add almond flour, salt and water into a saucepan. Place the saucepan over medium heat.
2. Stir constantly until thick.
3. Turn off the heat. Add cheese and stir until cheese melts.
4. Ladle into bowls and serve hot.

Comforting Keto Grits

Serves: 4

Ingredients:

- 4 cups cauliflower rice (cauliflower grated to rice like texture)
- 1 teaspoon salt
- ½ cup hemp hearts
- 4 ounces shredded cheddar cheese
- 2 cups unsweetened milk of your choice or more
- ½ teaspoon garlic powder
- ½ teaspoon pepper
- 4 tablespoons butter
- ½ cup heavy cream

Directions:

1. Place a cast iron skillet over medium-low heat. Add butter. When butter melts, add cauliflower and hemp hearts and stir-fry for a couple of minutes.
2. Stir in milk, cream, salt, pepper and garlic powder. Cook until thick and cauliflower is soft. Add more milk if required. You can also add water.
3. Turn off the heat. Add cheddar cheese and stir. Taste and adjust the seasoning if required.
4. Ladle into bowls and serve hot.

Keto Shrimp and Cauliflower "Grits"

Serves: 8

Ingredients:

- 2 medium cauliflowers, grated to rice like texture
- ½ cup water
- 2 pounds raw shrimp, peeled, deveined, discard tails
- Salt to taste
- Pepper to taste
- 4 tablespoons olive oil, divided
- 4 cups shredded cheddar cheese
- 4 teaspoons Cajun seasoning or to taste
- 2 tablespoons chopped parsley or cilantro or scallions

Directions:

1. Place a large pot over medium heat. Add 2 tablespoons oil. When the oil is heated, add cauliflower and water and cook until cauliflower is tender. Stir often.
2. Add cheese, salt and pepper and mix well. Turn off the heat.
3. Sprinkle Cajun seasoning, salt and pepper over the shrimp. Toss well.
4. Place a large skillet over medium heat. Add 2 tablespoons oil. When the oil is heated, add shrimp and cook for 2 – 3 minutes. Flip sides and cook the other side for 2 – 3 minutes.

5. Ladle grits into bowls. Top with shrimp. Sprinkle parsley on top and serve.

Breakfast Biscuit with Coconut Flour

Serves: 4

Ingredients:

- 4 tablespoons coconut flour
- ¼ teaspoon sea salt
- 4 teaspoons ghee or unsalted butter, cold
- ½ cup flaxseed meal
- 2 teaspoons baking powder
- 4 large eggs, beaten

Directions:

1. Add coconut flour, salt, flaxseed meal and baking powder into a bowl and stir.
2. Add ghee and mix well until crumbly. Add egg and mix well.
3. Grease 4 small oven proof bowls and divide the batter into the bowls.
4. Bake in a preheated oven at 350° F for 15 minutes or cook in a microwave on high for about 55 to 60 seconds.
5. Remove from the oven or microwave and place on a rack to cool.

Keto Biscuits

Serves: 4 – 5

Ingredients:

- ¾ cup super fine almond flour
- ½ tablespoon baking powder
- ¼ teaspoon onion powder
- ¼ teaspoon garlic powder
- 1/8 teaspoon salt
- 1 large egg
- 8 tablespoons butter, melted
- ¼ cup sour cream
- ¼ cup shredded cheddar cheese

Directions:

1. Grease a 6 counts muffin tin with some oil or butter.
2. Add almond flour, baking powder, onion powder, garlic powder and salt into a bowl and stir well.
3. Add eggs, butter and sour cream into a bowl and whisk until well incorporated.
4. Transfer into the bowl of almond flour.
5. Add cheese and stir.
6. Divide the batter into the prepared muffin tin.
7. Bake in a preheated oven at 450° F for 10 – 15 minutes or until a toothpick when inserted in the middle of biscuits comes out clean and the top is golden brown.
8. Remove from the oven and cool for a few minutes.

9. Serve warm.

Stuffed Breakfast Biscuits

Serves: 12

Ingredients:

- 4 ounces cream cheese
- 4 eggs, beaten
- Salt to taste
- Pepper to taste
- 12 breakfast sausage patties
- 4 cups shredded mozzarella cheese + extra to top
- 2 cups almond flour
- 4 ounces Colby Jack cheese thin cubes or any other variety of cheese

Directions:

1. Add cream cheese and mozzarella cheese into a microwave safe bowl. Microwave on High for 1-2 minutes or until cheese melts and the mixture well incorporated. Stir well every 30 seconds until the mixture melts and is smooth.
2. Add eggs into a bowl and whisk well. Add almond flour and mix well.
3. Stir in the cheese mixture and mix until well incorporated. Dough may be sticky.

4. Sprinkle some extra almond flour on the dough and shape into a ball. Wrap in plastic wrap and chill for 30-40 minutes.
5. Grease a 12 counts muffin tin with cooking spray.
6. Divide the dough into 12 equal portions and shape into balls.
7. Take one ball of dough and place it on your palm. Flatten the dough.
8. Place a sausage patty in the center of the dough and bring the edges together to enclose the patty.
9. Place in the muffin tin.
10. Repeat steps 7-9 and make the remaining biscuits.
11. Bake in a preheated oven at 350° F for 20-25 minutes or until golden brown. Sprinkle some more mozzarella on top and serve.

Southern Style Fluffy Biscuits

Serves: 10

Ingredients:

- ½ cup coconut flour
- 1 ½ cups almond flour
- 2 teaspoons baking powder
- ½ cup almond milk
- 10 egg whites
- ½ teaspoon sea salt
- 4 tablespoons butter or ghee + extra to brush on top of the biscuits

Directions:

1. Add coconut flour, almond flour, baking powder, and salt into a bowl and stir well.
2. Add almond milk and butter and stir until coarse crumbs are formed.
3. Set the electric hand mixer on high speed and whip until soft peaks are formed.
4. Pour into the bowl of dry ingredients. Set the hand mixer on low and mix until well incorporated.
5. Set aside for 5 minutes. If the batter is runny, add coconut flour, a little at a time and mix well each time. When the dough is ready, it should be thick.

6. Divide the dough into 10 equal portions and place on a baking sheet lined with parchment paper. Leave some gap between the biscuits.
7. Bake in a preheated oven at 350° F for 20 minutes or until golden brown. Brush with some butter half way through baking.

Southern Biscuits and Gravy

Serves: 5

Ingredients:

For biscuits:

- 1 ½ cups finely ground almond flour
- 1/8 teaspoon xanthan gum
- 1/8 teaspoon salt
- 1 egg
- ½ tablespoon baking powder
- ¼ teaspoon garlic powder
- 3 tablespoons butter, softened

For gravy:

- ½ pound ground breakfast sausage
- 1 ounce cream cheese, chopped
- ¼ cup chicken broth
- ¼ teaspoon pepper
- 1 tablespoon butter
- ¼ cup heavy whipping cream
- 1/8 teaspoon xanthan gum
- Salt to taste

Directions:

1. Add almond flour, xanthan gum, salt, baking powder and garlic powder into a mixing bowl and stir.

2. Stir in the butter and eggs and mix until well incorporated.
3. Divide the dough into 5 equal portions and shape into balls. Flatten the balls and place on a baking sheet lined with parchment paper.
4. Bake in a preheated oven at 400° F for 12 to 14 minutes or until they start to brown. Let it cool completely in the oven.
5. To make gravy: Place a skillet over medium heat. Add sausage and cook until it is not pink anymore. Break it simultaneously as it cooks.
6. Stir in butter and cream cheese and cook until cream cheese melts completely.
7. Add broth and cream and stir. Sprinkle xanthan gum on top and stir. Add pepper and stir. When it begins to bubble, remove from heat. Keep stirring until thick.
8. To serve: Place biscuits on individual serving plates. Spoon some gravy on top and serve.

Lowcountry Recipes

Keto Country Gravy

Serves: 8

Ingredients:

- 8 ounces breakfast sausage
- 2 cups heavy cream
- Salt to taste
- Pepper to taste
- 4 tablespoons butter
- 1 teaspoon guar gum

Directions:

1. Place a skillet over medium heat. Add sausage and cook until brown all over. Remove with a slotted spoon and place in a bowl.
2. Add butter into the skillet. When butter melts, stir in the cream.
3. Lower the heat to low heat and let the mixture come to a low boil.
4. Stir in the guar gum. Stir constantly until thick.
5. Add the browned sausage and mix well.
6. Turn off the heat and serve hot.

Chicken Shrimp Gumbo with Sausage

Serves: 4

Ingredients:

- 1 ½ tablespoons extra-virgin olive oil
- 2 cloves garlic, peeled, minced
- ½ green bell pepper, chopped
- ½ teaspoon sea salt
- Cayenne pepper to taste
- 1 can (14 ounces) crushed tomatoes
- 1 tablespoon butter
- 1 pound boneless chicken thighs, cubed
- 1 small onion, sliced
- 2 small stalks celery, chopped
- ½ teaspoon Cajun seasoning
- ½ tablespoon gumbo file powder
- 1 cup beef broth
- ½ pound shrimp, peeled, deveined
- 6 ounces Andouille sausage, thinly sliced

Directions:

1. Place a cast iron pot over medium-high heat. Add oil. When the oil is heated, add chicken and garlic and cook until chicken is brown.
2. Add bell pepper, onion and celery and stir. Cook until slightly soft.
3. Stir in the broth and tomatoes.

4. Lower the heat to medium heat and simmer for 3 – 4 minutes.
5. Stir in the butter and sausage. Lower the heat medium-low and cook for 15 minutes.
6. Add gumbo file powder and simmer for 2 minutes.
7. Stir in the shrimp and simmer for 3 minutes.
8. Ladle into bowls. Drizzle some hot sauce on top and serve.

Crab Deviled Eggs

Serves: 6

Ingredients:

- 6 hardboiled eggs, peeled, halved lengthwise
- ¼ cup keto friendly mayonnaise
- ½ tablespoon finely chopped celery
- 1 small green onion, finely chopped
- ½ tablespoon finely chopped green bell pepper
- ½ teaspoon minced fresh parsley + extra to garnish
- Pepper to taste
- Salt to taste
- ¼ teaspoon hot pepper sauce
- ½ can (from a 6 ounces can) crabmeat, drained, flaked, discard cartilage
- 1 teaspoon Dijon mustard
- ¼ teaspoon Worcestershire sauce

Directions:

1. Scoop out the yolks and place in a bowl. Set aside the whites.
2. Mash the yolks and add rest of the ingredients. Mix well.
3. Fill the whites with this mixture.
4. Cover and chill until use.
5. Garnish with parsley and serve.

Lowcountry Seafood Boil

Serves: 4

Ingredients:

- 2 gallons water
- 1 onion, quartered
- 1 ½ tablespoons salt
- 3 bay leaves
- 1 lemon halved
- 1 ½ tablespoons paprika or to taste
- 1 tablespoon ground allspice
- ½ tablespoon chili powder
- ½ tablespoon onion powder
- ½ tablespoon dry mustard
- ½ tablespoon dried thyme
- 1 ¼ teaspoons peppercorns
- 1 ½ tablespoons salt or to taste
- 2 teaspoons ground coriander
- ½ tablespoon chili powder
- ½ tablespoon garlic powder
- ½ tablespoon dried marjoram
- ½ tablespoon dried tarragon
- ½ tablespoon dried rosemary
- ½ teaspoon ground cumin
- 1 pound Italian sausage, cut into thirds
- 1 ¼ pounds cod fillets
- ¾ pound large raw shrimp, with shells

- ¾ pound mussels
- 1 ¾ pounds snow crab legs

Directions:

1. Pour water into a large stockpot. Place the pot over high heat.
2. When it begins to boil, add all the herbs, spices, onion, lemon and salt. Lower the heat and let it simmer.
3. Place a skillet over medium heat. Add sausage and cook until brown all over.
4. Remove sausage with a slotted spoon and place in a bowl. Discard extra fat from the skillet.
5. Add mussels into the skillet. Also add ½ cup of the simmering spiced water and stir.
6. Cover and cook for 5 minutes. If any mussels do not open, discard those. Turn off the heat.
7. Transfer into the stockpot. Add cod and sausage and stir.
8. Let it simmer for 5 minutes.
9. Stir in the crab legs and mussels. Let it simmer for 5 minutes.
10. Add shrimp and simmer until it turns pink. Turn off the heat.
11. Transfer the contents of the stockpot into a colander to drain. Add the contents of the colander into a serving bowl.
12. Serve.

Keto Mississippi Roast

Serves: 4

Ingredients:

- 1.9 pound beef chuck roast
- ½ tablespoon dried parsley
- ½ tablespoon garlic powder
- ½ tablespoon dried dill
- ½ tablespoon dried chives
- ½ tablespoon onion powder
- 1/8 teaspoon pepper
- ¼ teaspoon salt
- 1 tablespoon better than bouillon
- ½ jar (from a 16 ounces jar) deli-sliced pepperoncini's, drained but retain about ½ cup brine
- ¼ cup chopped butter

Directions:

1. Place chuck roast in a roasting pan.
2. Scatter pepperoncini's on top of the roast. Pour the retained brine all around the brine.
3. Mix together all the spices, salt and herb in a bowl. Sprinkle this mixture all over the top of the roast. Also place better than bouillon paste.
4. Place butter pieces all over the roast.
5. Cover the pan tightly with foil. When you bake it, it goes this way – one hour of baking for every pound of the meat.

6. Bake in a preheated oven at 300° F for about 2 hours or until it can be shredded easily with a fork.
7. You can also make it in a slow cooker for 5 – 6 hours on high.
8. Shred the meat with a pair of forks.
9. Serve hot.

Keto Creamy Crab Soup

Serves: 4 – 5

Ingredients:

- 1 ½ tablespoons butter
- 1 ounce cream cheese
- 8 ounces half and half
- 1 teaspoon Old Bay seafood seasoning
- ½ tablespoon chopped chives
- 1 ½ tablespoons almond flour
- 1 cup heavy whipping cream
- 7.5 ounces canned crab or ½ pound crab
- ¼ teaspoon keto friendly Creole seasoning or more to taste (optional)
- Grated Parmesan cheese, to serve (optional)

Directions:

1. Place a pot over medium-low heat. Add butter. When butter melts, add almond flour and cream cheese and stir until well combined.
2. Add whipping cream and half and half and whisk until well combined.
3. Add rest of the ingredients and stir. Lower the heat to medium-low heat and heat thoroughly.
4. Ladle into soup bowls. Garnish with Parmesan cheese and serve.

Southern Summer Tomato Pie

Serves: 12

Ingredients:

For crust:

- 1 ½ cups almond flour
- 2 eggs
- 4 tablespoons butter or coconut oil
- 2/3 cup oat fiber
- ½ teaspoon salt
- 2 eggs

For filling:

- 10 large tomatoes, sliced
- 1 cup keto friendly mayonnaise
- 2/3 cup finely sliced red onions
- 2 cups shredded cheese
- ½ teaspoon dried oregano, or more if required
- ½ teaspoon dried basil, or more if required

Directions:

1. Add all the ingredients for crust into a bowl and mix well.
2. Divide the dough into 2 pie pans (9 inches each). Spread it onto the bottom and the sides of the pie pan. Press it well.

3. Bake in a preheated oven at 350° F for 12 to 14 minutes or until they start to brown. Remove from the oven and let it cool.
4. Lay the tomato slices over the crusts. Make one or 2 layers of the tomatoes. Use all the tomatoes to layer the crusts.
5. Layer with onion slices.
6. Add mayonnaise and cheese into another bowl and stir. Spread the mixture over the onion layer. The onions and tomatoes should not be visible.
7. Sprinkle oregano and basil on top.
8. Bake in a preheated oven at 350° F for about 30minutes or until brown on top.
9. Remove from the oven and let it rest for 10 minutes.
10. Cut into wedges and serve.

Cajun Shrimp Boil

Serves: 8

Ingredients:

- 2 pounds large shrimp, peeled, deveined
- 4 medium zucchinis, sliced
- 28 ounces Andouille sausage, sliced
- 4 medium yellow squash, sliced
- 4 tablespoons olive oil
- Salt to taste
- 4 tablespoons Cajun seasoning
- Pepper to taste

Directions:

1. Place all the vegetables, sausage and shrimp on a sheet pan.
2. Sprinkle the seasoning, salt and pepper and toss well.
3. Drizzle oil and mix until well coated. Spread it evenly.
4. Bake in a preheated oven at 350° F for about 15 – 20 minutes or until shrimp turns pink.
5. Stir and serve.

Lowcountry-style Shrimp and Grits

Serves: 4

Ingredients:

<u>For grits:</u>

- ½ cup water
- 6 tablespoons blanched almond flour
- ¼ teaspoon salt
- Pepper to taste
- ¼ cup cheddar cheese (optional)
- 2 tablespoons unsalted butter
- 2 tablespoons coconut flour
- ¼ teaspoon garlic powder
- 1 ½ cups cooked cauliflower rice
- 2 ounces cream cheese

<u>For shrimp and gravy:</u>

- 1 tablespoon avocado oil
- 1 small white onion, diced
- 2 teaspoons minced garlic
- 1 tablespoon lemon juice
- ½ green bell pepper, diced
- ½ teaspoon dried oregano
- ½ teaspoon smoked paprika
- 1 teaspoon Old Bay seasoning

- 1 pound large shrimp, peeled, deveined, thaw and drain if frozen
- 2 ounces chicken broth
- ½ can (14.5 ounces each) diced tomatoes, drained
- Salt to taste
- Pepper to taste
- ½ tablespoons chopped fresh parsley

Directions:

1. To make grits: Add water and butter into a saucepan. Place the saucepan over medium-high heat. When butter melts, add coconut flour, almond flour, garlic powder, salt and pepper and stir constantly until slightly thick.
2. Stir in the cauliflower and cheddar cheese. Heat thoroughly. Turn off the heat.
3. Add cream cheese and mix well. Cover and set aside until the gravy is prepared.
4. To make gravy: Place a nonstick pan over medium-high heat. Add oil. When the oil is heated, add onion, lemon juice, bell pepper, garlic, spices and dried herbs. Cook until slightly tender.
5. Stir in the shrimp and toss well. Cook until shrimp is slightly pink on the edges.
6. Stir in tomatoes, salt and chicken broth and cook for a couple of minutes until the shrimp turn pink.
7. Add parsley and stir. If you find that the gravy is runny, take out the shrimp and set aside. Cook until the gravy is thicker. Add the shrimp and stir.

8. Divide grit into bowls. Top with shrimp and gravy and serve.

Low Country Shrimp Frittata

Serves: 2 – 3

Ingredients:

- 1 tablespoon extra-virgin olive oil
- ¼ cup chopped onion
- ¼ cup chopped celery
- 2 tablespoons milk of your choice
- Salt to taste
- Freshly ground pepper to taste
- 1 tablespoon chopped fresh flat leaf parsley
- 5 large eggs
- ½ cup cooked, chopped shrimp
- ½ teaspoon seafood seasoning or to taste

Directions:

1. Place an ovenproof skillet (small size) over medium-high heat. Add ½ tablespoon oil. When the oil is heated, add onion, celery and green bell pepper and sauté until lightly soft.
2. Remove the vegetables onto a plate.
3. Add eggs, salt, pepper and milk into a bowl and whisk well.
4. Add shrimp, seafood seasoning, parsley and the sautéed vegetables and mix well.
5. Add remaining oil into the skillet. When the oil is heated, add the egg mixture and spread it all over the pan. Let it

cook for a couple of minutes. Turn off the heat and place in the oven.
6. Bake in a preheated oven at 400° F for about 15 – 20 minutes. Remove from the oven and let it rest for a few minutes.
7. Cut into wedges and serve.

Keto Dogs

Serves: 3

Ingredients:

- 1 cup shredded mozzarella cheese
- 1 large egg, beaten
- 1 teaspoon baking powder
- 4 hot dogs
- ½ teaspoon garlic powder
- Mustard, to serve
- 2 ounces cream cheese
- 1 ¼ cups almond flour
- ½ teaspoon kosher salt
- 2 tablespoons butter, melted
- ½ tablespoon chopped fresh parsley

Directions:

1. Place a sheet of parchment paper on a baking sheet.
2. Add cream cheese and mozzarella cheese into a microwave safe bowl. Microwave for high for 40 – 50 seconds or until it melts. Stir every 15 seconds.
3. Stir in the eggs.
4. Stir in the almond flour, salt and baking powder.
5. Divide the mixture into 4 equal portions and shape into long log.
6. Wrap each hot dog with one log.
7. Add butter, parsley and garlic powder into a bowl and stir.

8. Brush this mixture over the hot dogs. Place on the baking sheet.
9. Bake in a preheated oven at 400° F for about 15 minutes or until golden brown.
10. Remove from the oven and let it cool for 5 minutes before serving.
11. Drizzle some mustard on top and serve.

Floribbean Recipes

Jamaican-Style Brown Chicken Stew

Serves: 8

Ingredients:

- 2 whole chickens, cut into pieces
- 4 carrots, peeled, sliced
- 2 red onions, chopped
- 4 tablespoons minced, fresh ginger
- 4 bell peppers, diced
- 7 – 8 green onions, sliced
- 6 cloves garlic, minced
- 2 scotch bonnet peppers or any other pepper, minced
- Juice from 2 limes
- 2 teaspoons smoked paprika
- 4 tablespoons coconut aminos
- 1 cup chicken stock
- Freshly ground pepper to taste
- Salt to taste
- 4 teaspoons minced fresh thyme
- 4 teaspoons ground allspice
- 4 cups coconut milk
- 2 tablespoons ghee or coconut oil or more if required

Directions:

1. Add green and red onions, garlic, peppers, paprika, garlic, thyme, ginger, salt, pepper and coconut aminos into a large bowl and stir well.
2. Add chicken into it and stir until chicken is well coated. Cover and refrigerate for 2 – 12 hours.
3. Place a Dutch oven over high heat. Add ghee. When ghee melts, add only the chicken pieces (retain the marinade) and cook until brown all over. Cook in batches if required.
4. Add the marinade and stir.
5. Lower the heat to medium heat and stir in the carrots and bell peppers.
6. Add stock and stir. Scrape the bottom of the pot to remove any browned bits that may be stuck.
7. Add coconut milk and mix well. Cover and cook until chicken is tender.
8. Turn off the heat.
9. Ladle into soup bowls and serve.

Jamaican Callaloo

Serves: 6

Ingredients:

- 8 cups callaloo
- 1 large onion, chopped
- 4 green onions, chopped
- 2 medium tomatoes, chopped
- 2 Scotch Bonnet peppers or ½ teaspoon cayenne pepper
- 2 tablespoons olive oil or coconut oil
- 4 cloves garlic, peeled, minced
- 4 sprigs thyme
- Salt to taste
- 4 tablespoons water

Directions:

1. Remove the membranes from the stalks of callaloo leaves. Discard the old leaves.
2. Place callaloo in a bowl of cold water with a teaspoon of salt in it. Set aside for a while. Drain and rinse with fresh water. Drain and chop into smaller pieces.
3. Place a large pot over medium heat. Add oil. When the oil is heated, add rest of the ingredients except salt and callaloo and cook until onion turns pink.
4. Stir in callaloo, salt and 4 tablespoons water. Cook until tender.
5. Serve hot.

Callaloo and Saltfish

Serves: 4

Ingredients

- 2 pounds callaloo leaves, rinsed, chopped
- 2 sprigs thyme
- 1 pound saltfish (cod fish)
- 2 cloves garlic, crushed or 4 teaspoons garlic powder
- 2 scotch bonnet peppers
- Pepper to taste
- ½ cup water
- 2 tablespoons margarine or vegetable oil
- 1 large onion, chopped
- Salt to taste

Directions:

1. Place a skillet over medium heat. Add oil. When the oil is heated, add saltfish, garlic, thyme, onion and pepper and sauté until onions are translucent.
2. Add callaloo leaves and water and mix.
3. Cover with a lid and cook until tender.
4. Add scotch bonnet pepper, salt and pepper. Simmer for a few minutes.
5. Serving options: Serve with avocado slices if desired.

Jerk Prawns

Serves: 8

Ingredients:

- 1 cup minced onion
- 12 cloves garlic, minced
- 8-10 scotch bonnet chilies or more to taste
- 1 teaspoon ground nutmeg
- ½ teaspoon ground cinnamon
- 4 teaspoons whole pimento
- ½ cup vegetable oil
- ½ cup water
- 2 teaspoons salt
- ½ cup chopped spring onions
- 2 tablespoons minced ginger
- 4 teaspoons minced fresh thyme
- 10 whole cloves
- 2 tablespoons swerve brown sugar
- 6 bay leaves
- ½ cup vinegar
- ½ teaspoon black pepper
- 4 pounds prawns

Directions:

1. To make jerk prawns: Add all the ingredients of jerk prawns except prawns into a food processor and blend until smooth.

2. Place prawns in a bowl. Pour the mixture over it. Coat the prawns well. Let it marinate for a while.
3. Set an outdoor grill or BBQ to preheat over medium heat setting.
4. Brush oil over the grill grates. Place prawns on the preheated grill. Cook for 2-3 minutes. Flip sides and cook the other side for 2-3 minutes. Baste with the marinade while grilling.
5. Serve over cauliflower rice.

Grilled Hogfish Snapper with Old Bay Compound Butter

Serves: 8

Ingredients:

- 8 hogfish fillets
- Juice of 4 lemons
- Zest of 2 lemons, grated
- 2 lemons, thinly sliced
- 4 tablespoons Old Bay seasoning
- 1 cup butter, softened

Directions:

1. Set up a grill for direct heating and preheat it to medium-high.
2. To make compound butter: Add lemon juice, lemon zest, butter and Old bay seasoning into a bowl. Blend until well combined.
3. Place a sheet of foil on a baking sheet. Grease with cooking spray. Place the fish fillets on the baking sheet. Place about a tablespoon of butter on each fillet.
4. Grill for 7 – 8 minutes or until it flakes easily when pierced with a fork.

Low Carb Keto Arroz Con Pollo (Spanish rice with Chicken)

Serves: 3

Ingredients:

For chicken breasts:

- 1 pound skinless, boneless chicken breast
- ½ teaspoon salt
- ¼ teaspoon ground cumin
- ½ tablespoon extra-virgin olive oil
- ¼ teaspoon pepper or to taste
- ¼ teaspoon paprika

For Spanish rice:

- ½ tablespoon extra-virgin olive oil
- ¼ cup small diced yellow bell pepper
- ¼ cup diced onion
- ¼ cup small diced red bell pepper
- 2 cloves garlic, minced
- ½ jalapeño pepper, minced
- ½ tablespoon chili powder
- ½ teaspoon salt
- ¼ teaspoon pepper or to taste
- ¼ cup tomato sauce
- ½ teaspoon ground cumin

- ½ teaspoon dried oregano
- 12 ounces cauliflower rice, fresh or frozen

Directions:

1. Brush the chicken with some of the oil and place in a baking dish.
2. Add all the spices into a bowl and stir. Sprinkle all over the chicken.
3. Bake in a preheated oven at 450° F for about 15 to 18 minutes or until cooked through.
4. Remove the chicken from the oven and cover loosely with foil. Let it sit for 10 minutes.
5. Cut into slices of ½ inch width.
6. Place a skillet over medium heat. Add remaining oil. When the oil is heated, add onion, jalapeño and bell peppers and cook until slightly tender.
7. Stir in the garlic and cook for a few seconds until aromatic.
8. Stir in the spices and cook for 40 – 50 seconds.
9. Add cauliflower and cook until slightly tender.
10. Taste and adjust the seasoning if required.
11. Stir in tomato sauce.
12. Divide cauliflower rice into plates. Place chicken slices on top and serve.

Ajiaco

Serves: 3

Ingredients:

- 1 ½ tablespoons avocado oil
- ¼ cup diced carrots
- 2 cloves garlic, peeled, minced
- 1 medium onion, diced
- ¼ cup diced celery stalks
- 1 bay leaf
- ½ teaspoon pepper
- ½ teaspoon salt or to taste
- ½ teaspoon dried oregano
- ½ teaspoon dried parsley
- ½ teaspoon ground cumin
- ½ pound ham hocks
- 10 ounces skinless, boneless chicken thighs
- ½ cup unsweetened pumpkin puree
- ½ cup cauliflower florets
- ¼ cup halved radishes
- 1 ½ cups chicken broth
- Lemon wedges, to serve

Directions:

1. Place a pot over medium heat. Add oil. When the oil is heated, add onion, celery, carrot, bay leaf and garlic and cook until slightly tender.

2. Add all the spices, ham hocks and chicken and mix well.
3. Cook until chicken is light brown. Stir frequently.
4. Stir in the pumpkin puree and bone broth.
5. When it begins to simmer, add radish and cauliflower. Lower the heat to low heat.
6. Cover and simmer for 30 – 40 minutes or until the meat is coming off the ham hocks.
7. Remove the ham hock bones. Shred the chicken with a pair of forks. Discard bay leaf.
8. Mix well. Serve with lime wedges.

Jerk Chicken

Serves: 3

Ingredients:

- 1 ¾ pounds bone-in chicken pieces, pat dried
- 2 large cloves garlic, peeled
- ½ cup chopped green onions
- ½ inch ginger, peeled, sliced
- ½ habanero pepper
- ½ teaspoon salt
- ¼ teaspoon ground cumin
- 1 tablespoon ground allspice
- ¼ teaspoon ground cinnamon
- ¼ teaspoon ground nutmeg

- ¼ teaspoon ground cloves
- 1 tablespoon extra-virgin olive oil
- 2 tablespoon lime juice
- Cauliflower rice to serve
- Lime wedges, to serve
- ½ tablespoon swerve

Directions:

1. Set aside the chicken, lime wedges and cauliflower rice and add rest of the ingredients into a blender and blend until smooth.
2. Place chicken in a baking dish. Spoon the blended mixture all over the chicken. Place the chicken in a single layer in the baking dish.
3. Chill for 1 – 8 hours. Remove the chicken from the refrigerator 30 minutes before grilling.
4. Set an outdoor grill or BBQ to preheat over medium heat setting.
5. Brush oil over the grill grates. Place chicken on the preheated grill. Cook for 8 – 10 minutes. Flip sides and cook the other side for 8 - 10 minutes or until cooked through. Baste with the marinade while grilling.
6. You can also bake in an oven or cook in a grill pan.
7. Serve over cauliflower rice with lime wedges.

Jerk Chicken Salad

Serves: 6

Ingredients

- 1 pound Jerk chicken, boneless, skinless – refer the previous recipe
- 1 head romaine lettuce, chopped
- 3 stalks celery, sliced
- 1 ripe avocado, peeled, pitted, sliced
- ¼ cup mayonnaise
- 3 fire roasted red peppers, chopped
- 1 small English cucumber, sliced
- Salt to taste
- Pepper to taste

Directions:

1. Add all the ingredients into a bowl and toss well.
2. Cover and chill until use.

Jamaican Chicken Curry

Serves: 8

Ingredients

For Jamaican curry powder:

- 2 tablespoons cumin seeds
- 2 tablespoons fenugreek seeds
- 2 tablespoons black peppercorns
- 1 teaspoons whole allspice
- 2 tablespoons mustard seeds
- 2 tablespoons anise seeds
- 2 tablespoons coriander seeds
- 2 tablespoons turmeric powder

For Jamaican chicken curry:

- 6 tablespoons vegetable oil
- Coarse salt to taste
- Freshly ground pepper to taste
- 8 cloves garlic, minced
- 1 medium scotch bonnet pepper, minced
- 4 tablespoons fresh thyme, chopped
- 4 cups coconut milk
- 8 chicken legs, skinless, split
- 4 medium onions, thinly sliced
- 1 ½ tablespoon ginger, minced
- 8 tablespoons Jamaican curry powder or to taste

- 6 cups chicken stock
- Juice of a lime

Directions:

1. To make Jamaican curry powder: Place a skillet over medium heat. Add cumin, fenugreek, mustard, coriander seeds, black peppercorns and allspice. Roast until aromatic. Turn off the heat. Set aside to cool.
2. When cooled, transfer into a spice grinder and grind until fine. Add into a bowl. Add turmeric powder and stir well. Use as much as required and store the remaining in an airtight container.
3. To make chicken curry: Sprinkle salt and pepper over the chicken.
4. Place a Dutch oven over high heat. Add oil. When the oil is heated, add chicken and cook until brown all over. Do not crowd the chicken. Cook in batches if required.
5. Remove the chicken with a slotted spoon and place on a plate lined with paper towels.
6. Add onions, chili pepper, garlic and ginger into the pot. Cook until onion is soft.
7. Stir in thyme and curry powder and sauté for a few seconds until fragrant.
8. Add lime juice and stir. Add the chicken back into the pot. Pour stock and coconut milk.
9. When it begins to boil, lower the heat and cover the pot partially. Simmer until the chicken is coming off the bone. It may take 1-1 ½ hours. Remove any fat that floats on top if desired.

Jamaican Meat Pies or Patties

Serves: 6

Ingredients:

For the filling:

- ¼ pound 85% lean ground beef
- ¼ pound ground pork
- ½ small onion, chopped
- ¼ cup water
- 1 tablespoon butter
- ½ teaspoon Jamaican curry powder – previous recipe
- 1 teaspoon ground coriander
- ¼ teaspoon ground allspice
- A pinch ground cloves
- 1/8 teaspoon stevia powder
- ½ teaspoon dried thyme
- 1 teaspoon ground cumin
- ¼ teaspoon ground turmeric
- ½ teaspoon garlic powder
- Salt to taste
- Pepper to taste

For crust:

- 3 ounces cream cheese, softened
- ½ teaspoon turmeric powder
- 1/8 teaspoon stevia

- ¼ cup coconut flour
- 1 tablespoon cold water
- 2 tablespoons butter, softened
- A large pinch salt
- ¼ teaspoon baking powder
- ¾ cup milled flaxseed meal

Directions:

1. For filling: Add onion, scotch bonnet, garlic and water into a blender and blend until smooth.
2. Place a skillet over medium heat. Add beef and pork and cook until it is not pink anymore. Break it simultaneously as it cooks.
3. Add the blended mixture, salt, pepper and mix well. Cook until dry. Turn off the heat.
4. To make crust: Add cream cheese and butter into a bowl. Beat with an electric hand mixer until light and creamy.
5. Add coconut flour, flax meal, salt, turmeric, baking powder and stevia into another bowl and mix well. Add into the bowl of cream cheese. Also add cold water and mix until dough is formed.
6. Divide the mixture into 6 equal portions and shape into balls.
7. Place a sheet of parchment paper on your countertop. Place a ball of dough on it. Place another sheet of parchment paper over it. Roll with a rolling pin until round of about 4 to 5 inches.

8. Place 1 – 2 tablespoons of the mixture on one half of the rolled dough. Fold the other half over the filling. Press the edges together to seal and place on a lined baking sheet.
9. Repeat steps 7 – 8 and make the remaining pies.
10. Bake in a preheated oven at 350° F for about 25 minutes or until golden brown.

Keto Cuban Pork (Lechón)

Serves: 10

Ingredients:

- 2 pounds pork shoulder
- ½ tablespoon ground cumin
- ½ teaspoon pepper
- ¼ teaspoon cayenne pepper
- ½ tablespoon dried oregano
- ½ tablespoon paprika
- 1 ½ teaspoons sea salt
- 1 onion, coarsely chopped
- 2 tablespoons lemon juice
- 1 bay leaf
- 4 cloves garlic, minced
- 2 tablespoons white vinegar
- Cooked cauliflower rice to serve

Directions:

1. Add all the ingredients except cauliflower rice into a Dutch oven.
2. Place over low heat. Cook until pork is tender. Drain and shred with a pair of forks. Place on a baking sheet.
3. Set the oven to broil mode. Broil the pork until crisp.
4. Serve hot over cauliflower rice.

Keto Cuban Sliders

Serves: 4 – 6

Ingredients:

- 1 pound Swiss cheese
- 1 pound pulled pork
- 12 tablespoons unsalted butter
- 4 large pickles, sliced
- 1 pound uncured deli ham
- ¼ cup minced white onion
- 4 tablespoons yellow mustard
- 4 – 6 keto dinner rolls, split

Directions:

1. Spread butter on the cut part of the dinner rolls. Layer with cheese, pork, onion, ham, pickles and mustard. Cover with the top half of the rolls.
2. Bake in a preheated oven at 350° F for a few minutes until cheese melts.

Keto Cuban Cups

Serves: 12

Ingredients:

- 12 medium slices salami
- 6 teaspoons Dijon mustard
- 3 ounces pickles, chopped
- 3 slices cheese, quartered (square pieces)

Directions:

1. Take a 12 counts muffin pan. Place a slice of salami into each cup.
2. Divide the pickles among the cups. Place ½ teaspoon mustard in each cup.
3. Place a piece of cheese in each cup.
4. Bake in a preheated oven at 350° F for about 12 – 15 minutes or until the edges are crisp. Remove from the oven and let it rest for a few minutes.

Puerto Rican Chicken

Serves: 8

Ingredients:

- 4 pounds chicken drumsticks
- 4 tablespoons chili powder
- 2 tablespoons coriander seeds, crushed
- 2 packages cauliflower rice (about 8 cups)
- 1 ½ cups roasted red peppers
- 1 cup avocado oil
- 4 tablespoons granulated onions
- 4 cups packed cilantro
- 4 tablespoons garlic powder
- 1 cup green olives
- 4 tablespoons capers
- Salt to taste

Directions:

1. Mix together chili powder and coriander in a bowl. Rub this mixture all over the chicken.
2. Cook the cauliflower rice according to the instructions on the package.
3. Place a large skillet over medium heat. Add a little oil. When the oil is heated, chicken and cook until brown all over. Remove chicken with a slotted spoon and set aside on a plate.

4. Add 1 cup roasted red peppers, cilantro, granulated onion, garlic and remaining avocado oil into a blender. Blend until smooth.
5. Pour into the skillet. Also add cauliflower rice and mix well. Add chicken and mix well.
6. Divide into plates. Garnish with olives, capers and remaining roasted red peppers and stir.

Caribbean Callaloo Soup

Serves: 10 – 12

Ingredients:

- 2 bunches callaloo leaves
- 2 tablespoons olive oil
- 8 cloves garlic, peeled, minced
- 2 whole scotch bonnet peppers, deseeded, chopped
- 2 teaspoons pepper or to taste
- 2 teaspoons salt or to taste
- 2 cups cubed pumpkin (small cubes)
- 2 cups vegetable stock
- 2 cups coconut milk
- 20 stalks okra, cut into 1 inch pieces
- ½ cup diced onions
- 2 large red bell peppers, chopped
- 2 teaspoons kosher salt
- 2 tablespoons smoked sweet paprika
- 6 sprigs fresh thyme
- 6 cups water

Directions:

1. Place a large soup pot over medium heat. Add oil. When the oil is heated, add onions and sauté until translucent.
2. Stir in the peppers and garlic and sauté for a couple of minutes.
3. Stir in the okra and pumpkin. Cook for 3 – 4 minutes.

4. Add rest of the ingredients and mix well. Simmer until vegetables are tender.
5. Ladle into soup bowls and serve

Caribbean Callaloo and Crab

Serves: 4

Ingredients:

- 9 taro leaves
- 1 medium onion, chopped
- 3 cloves garlic, crushed
- ¼ cup peeled, cubed pumpkin
- 1 small habanero pepper
- 2 blue crabs, cleaned, chopped
- 2 green onions, chopped
- 6 pods okra, finely chopped
- 2 sprigs fresh thyme
- 2 ounces salted pig's tail (optional)
- ½ cup water
- 1 ½ cups coconut milk
- Salt to taste

Directions:

1. Discard the skin from the stalks of taro leaves also discard the tip from the central rib. Wash well and chop into bite size pieces.
2. Add all the ingredients except crab and salt into a pot. Place the pot over low heat. Cover and cook until tender.
3. Add crab and cook for some more time until crab is cooked. Discard the habanero.

4. Add salt and stir. Blend with an immersion blender until smooth.
5. Serve over hot cauliflower rice.

Southern Dessert Recipes

Southern Butter Keto Pound Cake

Serves: 12

Ingredients:

- 6 large eggs
- ½ cup butter
- 4 teaspoons coconut flour
- 2 cups blanched almond flour
- ½ cup granulated sweetener
- ½ teaspoon baking powder
- 1 teaspoon butter extract
- ½ teaspoon salt
- 1 teaspoon liquid stevia or liquid monk fruit

Directions:

1. Grease a Bundt cake pan with a little oil or butter. Set aside.
2. Melt the butter and let it cool to room temperature.
3. Add all the dry ingredients to a bowl.
4. Add eggs and sweetener to a large mixing bowl. Beat with an electric mixer until well combined.
5. Add the dry ingredients into the mixing bowl at a time and beat until well combined.

6. Add butter extract and beat again.
7. Pour into the prepared dish.
8. Bake in a preheated oven 350° F for about 30 minutes or until a toothpick when inserted in the center comes out clean.
9. Cool for a while. Slice and serve.

Chocolate Cake

Serves: 12

Ingredients:

- ½ cup coconut flour
- ¾ cup swerve or erythritol
- 1 teaspoon baking powder
- 1 teaspoon baking soda
- ½ teaspoon ground cinnamon
- 1/8 teaspoon stevia concentrated powder
- ½ cup cocoa powder, unsweetened
- ¼ teaspoon sea salt
- 4 large eggs, beaten
- 2 cups shredded zucchini
- ¼ cup melted coconut oil
- 1 teaspoon vanilla extract
- 6 tablespoons sugar-free chocolate chips (optional)

For chocolate buttercream frosting: Optional

- ½ cup butter, softened
- 1/3 cup cocoa powder, unsweetened
- 1 teaspoon vanilla extract
- ½ cup swerve confectioners' or Sukrin Melis
- 2 tablespoons unsweetened almond milk or coconut milk or more if required
- ½ teaspoon stevia Glycerite or monk fruit powder

Directions:

1. To make cake: Add all the dry ingredients into a mixing bowl and stir.
2. Add all the wet ingredients except zucchini and chocolate chips if using, into the bowl of dry ingredients and whisk well.
3. Add zucchini and chocolate chips and fold gently.
4. Grease a small baking dish (6 inches) with cooking spray. Place a sheet of parchment paper.
5. Pour the batter into the dish.
6. Bake in a preheated oven at 350° F for about 25 minutes or a toothpick when inserted in the center comes out clean. Remove from the oven and set aside to cool for a while.
7. To make chocolate buttercream frosting: Add butter into a mixing bowl. Beat with an electric hand mixer until creamy. Add sweetener and cocoa and mix until creamy.
8. Add almond milk and beat until well combined.
9. Add stevia and vanilla and beat well.
10. Place the cake on a serving platter or cake stand. Spread the frosting over the cake. Refrigerate until use.
11. Cut into slices and serve.

Keto Southern Coconut Pecan Cake

Serves: 8 – 10

Ingredients:

For cake:

- 6 large eggs, separated
- 6 tablespoons solid coconut oil + extra to grease
- 1 ½ teaspoons vanilla extract
- 1 ½ teaspoons coconut extract
- 6 tablespoons coconut flour
- 1/8 teaspoon xanthan gum
- 2 tablespoons shredded coconut, unsweetened
- 1 ½ teaspoons cream of tartar
- 6 tablespoons swerve
- ¼ +1/8 teaspoon baking soda
- 1/8 teaspoon sea salt

For frosting: Optional

- 6 ounces cream cheese, softened
- ½ cup coconut milk, unsweetened
- ½ teaspoon coconut extract
- ½ teaspoon vanilla extract
- ¼ cup butter, softened
- 2 cups swerve confectioners
- 6 tablespoons shredded coconut, unsweetened, to garnish
- ¼ cup chopped, toasted pecans, to garnish

Directions:

1. Grease a baking dish (8 inches) with oil. Place a sheet of parchment paper on the bottom of the dish.
2. Add egg whites and cream of tartar into a bowl. Beat with an electric hand mixer until stiff peaks are formed.
3. Add coconut oil into another bowl and whip lightly. Beat in the yolks.
4. Add coconut flour, xanthan gum, swerve, baking soda, salt, vanilla and coconut extract and beat until well combined.
5. Add shredded coconut and stir with a spatula. Add whites and fold gently,
6. Spoon the batter into the baking dish.
7. Bake in a preheated oven at 350° F for about 25 minutes or a toothpick when inserted in the center comes out clean. Remove from the oven and set aside to cool for a while.
8. To make icing: Add cream cheese, swerve and butter into a bowl and beat until creamy.
9. Add coconut milk, vanilla and coconut extract and beat until well combined.
10. Place the cake on a serving platter or cake stand. Spread the icing on the cake.
11. Sprinkle pecans and coconut on top.
12. Refrigerate until use.
13. Cut into slices and serve.

Pumpkin Pie

Serves: 4

Ingredients:

For crust:

- 1 ½ cups desiccated coconut
- 4 tablespoons Brain octane oil or ½ tablespoon melted ghee or coconut oil
- 1 tablespoon coconut cream
- ¼ - ½ tablespoon swerve or erythritol

For pumpkin filling:

- 1 ½ tablespoons coconut oil or ghee or butter, melted
- 1 teaspoon CollaGelatin
- 7.5 ounces steamed pumpkin or canned solid pumpkin puree
- 1 teaspoon vanilla extract
- A pinch ground clove or cardamom
- ¼ cup coconut cream
- 2 tablespoons water
- 1 ½ teaspoons ground Ceylon cinnamon
- A pinch salt

To serve:

- Keto vanilla ice cream or whipped coconut cream.

Directions:

1. To make crust: Add coconut into the food processor bowl. Process until very fine. Add rest of the ingredients for crust and process until well combined.
2. Place a sheet of parchment paper on the bottom of a 6-inch pie pan. Place the mixture in pan and press it well onto the bottom as well as the sides of the pan.
3. Freeze until firm.
4. To make filling: Add CollaGelatin and water in a bowl and stir until it dissolves completely. Set aside for 5-8 minutes.
5. Place a saucepan with coconut cream over low heat. Add CollaGelatin mixture. Stir frequently until it dissolves completely. Turn off the heat.
6. Transfer into a blender. Add rest of the ingredients for filling and blend until smooth.
7. Spread the filling over the crust. Cover the pan with cling wrap and freeze for about 2 hours.
8. Cut into wedges and serve with keto vanilla ice cream or whipped coconut cream.

Keto Apple Pie

Serves: 8

Ingredients:

For crust:

- ¼ cup butter
- 6 tablespoons coconut flour
- ½ tablespoon whole psyllium husks
- ¾ cup almond flour
- 2 eggs
- ¼ teaspoon salt

For filling:

- 5 small chayote squashes, peeled, sliced
- ¾ teaspoon ground cinnamon
- A pinch ground nutmeg
- 1/8 teaspoon ground ginger
- ½ tablespoon xanthan gum
- ½ tablespoon lemon juice
- 3 tablespoons cold butter, cut into pieces
- 6 tablespoons swerve or erythritol + extra to sprinkle
- 1 teaspoon apple extract (optional)
- 1 small egg, beaten, to brush

Directions:

1. To make crust: Melt the butter and let it cool to room temperature: Add all the ingredients for crust including butter into a mixing bowl and mix well into dough.
2. Divide the dough into 2 equal portions and shape into balls.
3. Take a 5 – 6 inches pie pan. Place one ball of dough in it. Press it onto the bottom as well as the sides of the pan. Set aside the other ball of dough.
4. Place chayote slices and water in a saucepan. Place saucepan over medium heat. Cook until chayote is tender. Drain.
5. Add the chayote back into the saucepan. Add spices, sweetener, lemon juice and apple extract and mix well.
6. Spread the chayote mixture on the crust. Place butter pieces all over the filling.
7. Roll the other ball of dough (place in between 2 sheets of parchment paper while rolling) into a circle (of the about 5 – 6 inches) and place over the filling. Press the edges of both the crusts together to seal.
8. Make a few small slits on the top of the pie (in the rolled dough). Lightly brush beaten egg all over the top crust.
9. Sprinkle some sweetener all over the crust if desired.
10. Bake in a preheated oven at 375° F for around 30 minutes or until golden brown on top.
11. Cool slightly. Cut into 8 equal slices and serve.

Vegan Keto Chocolate Pie

Serves: 6

Ingredients:

For crust:

- 6 tablespoons coconut flour
- ¼ cup coconut oil, melted
- A tiny pinch salt
- 1 tablespoon psyllium husk
- ¼ cup water

For filling:

- 1 ounce unsweetened chocolate or stevia sweetened chocolate, melted
- ½ cup coconut oil
- ½ teaspoon stevia (optional, to be used if using unsweetened chocolate)
- 2 cans (14.5 ounces each) full fat coconut milk
- 2 cups almond butter

Directions:

1. To make crust: Add water and coconut oil into a bowl. Add psyllium husk and mix well. Stir for about a minute.
2. Add coconut flour and salt and stir. Set aside for a couple of minutes or until the water has been absorbed.

3. Place the dough in a small pie pan (about 5 – 6 inches). Press it well onto the bottom as well as the sides of the pan.
4. Prick the crust at a few places with a fork.
5. Bake in a preheated oven at 350° F for around 30 minutes or until light golden brown on top. Remove from the oven and let it cool for 15 minutes.
6. To make filling: Add all the ingredients for filling into a blender and blend until well incorporated. Pour over the crust.
7. Refrigerate for 8-9 hours.
8. Slice and serve.

Berry Crisp

Serves: 12

Ingredients:

- 2 – 3 teaspoons powdered erythritol or swerve
- 5 – 6 cups berries

For topping:

- 3 cups almond meal or almond flour
- 1 cup butter, softened
- 2 teaspoons vanilla extract
- 4 tablespoons powdered swerve or erythritol
- 1 teaspoon ground cinnamon
- 1 cup chopped pecans

To serve:

- Heavy cream

Directions:

1. Spread the berries in a baking dish. Sprinkle sweetener over it.
2. For topping: Add almond meal, butter, vanilla, sweetener and cinnamon into a bowl and mix well.
3. Add pecans and stir well.
4. Spread the topping over the berries.

5. Bake in a preheated oven at 350° F for around 30 minutes or until light golden brown on top. Remove from the oven and let it cool for 15 minutes.
6. Top with heavy cream and serve.

Blackberry Cobbler

Serves: 4

Ingredients:

For filling:

- 2 cups blackberries
- ½ teaspoon lemon juice
- 2 tablespoons Monkfruit sweetener
- 1/8 teaspoon xanthan gum

For topping:

- ½ cup almond flour
- 1 ½ tablespoons Monkfruit sweetener
- 2 tablespoons butter, melted
- ¼ teaspoon ground cinnamon

Directions:

1. To make filling: Add all the ingredients for filling into a baking dish and stir until well combined.
2. To make topping: Add all the ingredients for topping into a bowl and mix until crumbly.
3. Scatter the topping over the berries.

4. Bake in a preheated oven at 350° F for around 30 minutes or until light golden brown on top. Remove from the oven and let it cool for at least 15 minutes.
5. Serve warm or cold with keto ice cream if desired.

Brownies

Serves: 15 - 18

Ingredients:

- 1 ½ cups almond flour
- 1 ½ cups chopped macadamia nuts
- 10 tablespoons salted butter
- 4 large eggs
- 2 teaspoons vanilla extract
- 1 ½ cups erythritol
- ½ cup coconut oil
- 6 tablespoons cocoa powder
- 3 teaspoons baking powder
- 2 teaspoons instant coffee

Directions:

1. Line large baking dish (9 x 12 inches) with parchment paper.
2. Add butter, coconut oil and erythritol into a mixing bowl. Beat with an electric hand mixer until creamy.
3. Beat in the eggs.
4. Add almond flour, cocoa, baking powder and coffee and mix well. Add vanilla and half the hazelnuts and stir well.
5. Pour the batter into the baking dish. Scatter remaining hazelnuts on top. Press lightly to adhere.

6. Bake in a preheated oven 350° F for about 16 – 20 minutes or until a toothpick when inserted in the middle comes out clean.
7. Remove from the oven. Let it cool on a wire rack for 15 minutes.
8. Cut into 15 - 18 equal pieces and serve.

Lime Fluff

Serves: 4 – 5

Ingredients:

For fluff:

- 4 ounces cream cheese, softened
- 2 ½ teaspoons grated, key lime zest
- 5 tablespoons powdered Monkfruit sweetener
- ¾ cup heavy whipping cream
- 1 ½ tablespoons key lime juice

For topping:

- 1 tablespoon powdered Monkfruit sweetener
- ¼ cup heavy whipping cream

Directions:

1. For fluff: Add heavy cream into a bowl and beat on medium speed until stiff peaks are formed.
2. Add cream cheese, lime juice, lime zest and sweetener into a bowl. Beat until smooth.
3. Add the whipped cream into the bowl of cream cheese and beat until well incorporated.
4. Transfer into a greased pan or individual serving bowls.
5. For topping: Add heavy cream and sweetener into a bowl and beat on medium speed until stiff peaks are formed.
6. Spoon over the fluff and chill for 8 – 9 hours.
7. Serve chilled.

Keto Churros

Serves: 6 – 8

Ingredients:

- 4 tablespoons coconut flour
- 6 tablespoons almond flour
- ¼ teaspoon xanthan gum
- ½ cup water
- 1 teaspoon stevia extract
- 1 small egg
- A tiny pinch salt
- ½ tablespoon coconut oil
- A large pinch ground cinnamon + extra to garnish

To serve: Optional

- Sugar-free chocolate syrup
- 1 teaspoon powdered swerve or erythritol or stevia

Directions:

1. Add coconut flour, almond flour, salt and xanthan gum into a bowl and stir.
2. Add water, cinnamon, stevia and coconut oil into a saucepan. Place the saucepan over medium heat.
3. When it begins to boil, turn off the heat. Let it cool for 3 to 4 minutes.
4. Stir in the dry ingredients with a rubber spatula.
5. Stir in the egg. Mix until well combined.

6. Transfer dough into a piping bag. Fit a star tip nozzle in the piping bag.
7. Place a sheet of parchment paper on a baking sheet.
8. Pipe the churros on the parchment. Choose the length of the churros that suits you.
9. Bake in a preheated oven 350° F for about 16 – 20 minutes until golden brown on the edges.
10. Set the oven to broil mode, on low and broil for a few minutes until golden brown.
11. Remove from the oven and cool for a few minutes. Sprinkle cinnamon and sweetener on top and serve with sugar-free chocolate syrup.

Conclusion

Thank you for purchasing the book.

If you are someone who has always loved Southern food, but has an issue with weight, you do not have to worry anymore. Southern cuisine is very unhealthy since it includes high-fat, high-carb and high-sugar ingredients. It is for this reason that most people wonder if they should continue to eat food from the Southern cuisine. They love the delicious food, but are worried that it will affect their health. Numerous studies show that Southern cuisine is terrible for overall health. That said, there is always a way to workaround this. All you need to do is find the ingredients you can use instead of high-carb ingredients.

If you want to follow the ketogenic diet and continue to eat the Southern cuisine, but do not know where to begin, you have come to the right place. This book has some delicious recipes that will help you ease into the Ketogenic diet while you continue to consume Southern food. These recipes are easy to make and extremely delicious. They will most definitely make your mouth water. I hope you enjoy the recipes in the book!

www.ingramcontent.com/pod-product-compliance
Lightning Source LLC
Chambersburg PA
CBHW070729020526
44107CB00077B/2266